Breathe Easy: A Comprehensive Guide to Allergy Relief

Welcome to "Breathe Easy: A Comprehensive Guide to Allergy Relief." This book is designed to provide you with the knowledge, strategies, and tools to effectively manage and find relief from allergies. Whether you suffer from seasonal allergies, food allergies, or environmental allergies, this book is your roadmap to a life of greater comfort and well-being.

The purpose of this book is to empower you with information about allergies and equip you with practical solutions to alleviate symptoms, prevent allergic reactions, and enhance your quality of life. Allergies can be disruptive and limit your daily activities, but with the right knowledge and approach, you can take control of your allergies and experience the freedom to live your life to the fullest.

Through this comprehensive guide, we will delve into the various aspects of allergies, including understanding their causes, identifying symptoms, seeking diagnosis, and exploring a range of treatment options. We will explore both natural remedies and medical treatments, helping you make informed decisions about what works best for you.

Additionally, we will address the emotional and social challenges that often accompany allergies and provide strategies to manage these aspects of your well-being. Our aim is not only to provide relief from physical symptoms but also to support your overall emotional health and resilience.

It's time to reclaim your life from the grip of allergies. This book is here to guide and empower you on your journey to allergy relief. Let's embark on this path together, arming ourselves with knowledge and implementing practical strategies to breathe easy and enjoy a life free from the constraints of allergies.

I. Understanding Allergies

- Definition of allergies
- Common types of allergies (seasonal, food, environmental, etc.)
- Causes and triggers of allergies
- The body's immune response to allergens

II. Allergy Symptoms and Diagnosis

- Common allergy symptoms
- Identifying and tracking allergy triggers
- Seeking medical diagnosis and testing

III. Managing Allergies through Lifestyle Changes

- Allergen avoidance strategies
- Creating an allergy-friendly home environment
- Tips for managing allergies at work and in public spaces
- Allergy-friendly travel tips

IV. Natural Remedies for Allergy Relief

- Herbal remedies and supplements
- Nasal rinses and saline sprays
- Breathing exercises and relaxation techniques
- Essential oils for allergy relief

V. Medical Treatments For Allergies

- Over-the-counter medications for symptom relief
- Prescription medications for allergies
- Allergy shots (immunotherapy)
- Alternative treatments (acupuncture, chiropractic care, etc.)

VI. Managing Allergies in Specific Scenarios

- Allergies in children and infants
- Allergies during pregnancy
- Allergies and aging
- Allergies and comorbid conditions (asthma, eczema, etc.)

VII. Allergy Prevention and Long-Term Management

- Strategies for preventing allergies
- Creating an allergy action plan
- Regular check-ups and monitoring
- Allergy support groups and resources

VIII. Dealing with Allergy Challenges and Emotional Well-being

- Coping with the emotional impact of allergies
- Overcoming challenges in social situations
- Self-care practices for managing allergies

- Seeking support and building resilience

IX. Conclusion

- Recap of allergy relief strategies
- Encouragement for readers on their allergy journey
- Final words of motivation and empowerment
- Additional resources and references for further exploration

I.Understanding Allergies

Definition Of Allergies

Allergies are a hypersensitive response of the immune system to substances that are typically harmless to most individuals. These substances, known as allergens, can trigger an immune reaction in susceptible individuals, leading to various symptoms and allergic reactions.

Allergens can include a wide range of substances, such as pollen, dust mites, pet dander, certain foods, insect venom, mold spores, and certain medications. When a person with allergies comes into contact with an allergen, their immune system produces an antibody called immunoglobulin E (IgE). The IgE antibodies bind to specific cells in the body, such as mast cells and basophils.

Upon subsequent exposure to the same allergen, the IgE antibodies trigger the release of various chemical mediators, including histamine, from these cells. Histamine is responsible for many of the symptoms associated with allergies, such as itching, swelling, sneezing, runny nose, watery eyes, hives, and in severe cases, difficulty breathing or anaphylaxis.

Allergies can range in severity, with some individuals experiencing mild symptoms, while others may have more severe and potentially life-threatening reactions. Allergy symptoms can affect different systems of the body, including the respiratory system, skin, gastrointestinal system, and cardiovascular system.

It's important for individuals with allergies to identify and avoid their specific allergens, and in some cases, they may require medical treatment or interventions, such as antihistamines, nasal sprays, epinephrine auto-injectors for emergencies, or immunotherapy (allergy shots).

It's worth noting that allergies can develop at any age, and some individuals may outgrow certain allergies over time, while others may develop new allergies later in life. It's always advisable for individuals with suspected allergies to seek medical evaluation and guidance from healthcare professionals for accurate diagnosis and appropriate management.

Common Types Of Allergies (Seasonal, Food, Environmental, Etc.)

Allergies can manifest in various forms and affect different aspects of a person's life. Here are some common types of allergies:

Seasonal Allergies: Also known as hay fever or allergic rhinitis, seasonal allergies occur during specific times of the year when certain plants release pollen into the air. Common triggers include tree pollen in the spring, grass pollen in the summer, and weed pollen in the fall. Symptoms may include sneezing, runny nose, itchy and watery eyes, nasal congestion, and throat irritation.

Food Allergies: Food allergies occur when the immune system reacts to specific proteins in certain foods. Common food allergens include peanuts, tree nuts, milk, eggs, fish, shellfish, wheat, and soy. Symptoms can range from mild to severe and may include hives, swelling, itching, gastrointestinal issues, breathing difficulties, and in severe cases, anaphylaxis.

Environmental Allergies: Environmental allergies refer to allergies triggered by substances in the environment, such as dust mites, pet dander, mold spores, and insect venom. Dust mite allergies are common and can cause symptoms like sneezing, nasal congestion, itchy eyes, and asthma symptoms. Pet allergies can be triggered by proteins found in pet saliva, urine, or dander, leading to similar symptoms. Mold spores and insect venom can also cause allergic reactions in susceptible individuals.

Drug Allergies: Some people may develop allergies to certain medications, such as antibiotics (e.g., penicillin), non-steroidal anti-inflammatory drugs (NSAIDs), or medications like aspirin. Drug allergies can range from mild skin reactions to more severe symptoms like hives, swelling, difficulty breathing, or anaphylaxis.

Skin Allergies: Skin allergies can be caused by contact with allergens such as certain metals (e.g., nickel), latex, cosmetics, fragrances, or certain plants like poison ivy or poison oak. Contact dermatitis is a common skin allergy characterized by redness, itching, and skin rash at the site of contact.

It's important to note that these are just a few examples of common types of allergies, and there are other specific allergens that can trigger allergic reactions in individuals. If you suspect you have allergies, it's best to consult with a healthcare professional or allergist for proper diagnosis and management.

Causes And Triggers Of Allergies

Allergies are triggered by the immune system's response to substances that are typically harmless to most people. The immune system mistakenly identifies these substances, known as allergens, as a threat and launches an immune response to protect the body. The specific causes and triggers of allergies can vary depending on the type of allergy. Here are some common causes and triggers:

Environmental Allergens: Environmental allergens include substances found in the environment, such as pollen, dust mites, pet dander, mold spores, and insect venom. These allergens can be inhaled, touched, or ingested, leading to allergic reactions in susceptible individuals.

Food Allergens: Food allergies are triggered by proteins in certain foods. Common food allergens include peanuts, tree nuts, milk, eggs, fish, shellfish, wheat, and soy. It's important to note that food intolerances, such as lactose intolerance, are different from food allergies as they do not involve the immune system.

Medications: Certain medications can cause allergic reactions in susceptible individuals. Antibiotics like penicillin, non-steroidal anti-inflammatory drugs (NSAIDs) like ibuprofen, and other medications can trigger allergic reactions ranging from mild skin rashes to severe anaphylaxis.

Insect Stings: Insect venom from bees, wasps, hornets, and fire ants can trigger allergic reactions in individuals who are allergic to these stings. The venom contains proteins that can cause an immune response, leading to localized or systemic allergic reactions.

Contact Allergens: Some people may develop allergic reactions when their skin comes into contact with certain substances, such as metals (e.g., nickel), latex, cosmetics, fragrances, or plants like poison ivy. These allergens can cause skin irritation, redness, itching, and rashes.

It's important to remember that individuals can have different allergic triggers, and what may cause an allergic reaction in one person may not affect another. Identifying and avoiding specific allergens is crucial in managing allergies. If you suspect you have allergies, it's recommended to consult with a healthcare professional or allergist for proper diagnosis, testing, and guidance on managing your allergies.

The Body's Immune Response To Allergens

When an allergen enters the body of an individual with allergies, the immune system recognizes it as a threat and initiates an immune response. This immune response involves several steps:

Sensitization: Upon initial exposure to an allergen, the immune system identifies it as foreign and starts producing specific antibodies called immunoglobulin E (IgE). These IgE antibodies bind to cells in the body known as mast cells and basophils, which are found in tissues such as the skin, respiratory tract, and digestive system.

Activation: In subsequent exposures to the same allergen, the allergen binds to the IgE antibodies already attached to the mast cells and basophils. This triggers the release of various chemicals, including histamine, leukotrienes, and cytokines, from these cells. Histamine, in particular, plays a significant role in causing allergy symptoms.

Inflammatory Response: The release of these chemicals leads to an inflammatory response in the body. Inflammation causes blood vessels to dilate, allowing more blood flow to the affected area. It also increases the permeability of blood vessels, leading to fluid leakage and swelling.

Allergic Symptoms: The immune response and inflammation caused by the release of chemicals can result in a wide range of allergic symptoms, depending on the type of allergen and the location of the immune response. Common symptoms include itching, sneezing, nasal congestion, runny nose, watery eyes, coughing, wheezing, hives, skin rashes, swelling, digestive issues, and in severe cases, anaphylaxis.

The severity and specific symptoms of an allergic reaction can vary from person to person and depend on factors such as the type of allergen, the route of exposure, the individual's sensitivity, and their overall health. It's important for individuals with allergies to be aware of their triggers, take precautions to avoid allergens, and seek appropriate medical care and treatment for managing their allergies.

II. Allergy Symptoms and Diagnosis

Common Allergy Symptoms

Allergy symptoms can vary depending on the type of allergy and the individual's response. Here are some common allergy symptoms:

Respiratory Symptoms:

- Sneezing
- Runny or stuffy nose (allergic rhinitis)
- Itchy or watery eyes (allergic conjunctivitis)
- Coughing
- Wheezing or shortness of breath (asthma)

Skin Symptoms:

- Itchy skin
- Hives (raised, red, itchy bumps on the skin)
- Eczema (red, itchy, and inflamed skin patches)
- Swelling (angioedema) of the lips, face, or other body parts

Gastrointestinal Symptoms:

- Abdominal pain or cramping
- Nausea or vomiting
- Diarrhea

Anaphylaxis (severe allergic reaction):

- Swelling of the throat, tongue, or lips
- Difficulty breathing or wheezing
- Rapid heartbeat
- Dizziness or fainting
- Confusion or disorientation
- Loss of consciousness

It's important to note that not all symptoms may occur in every individual with allergies, and the severity of symptoms can vary. Allergy symptoms typically occur shortly after exposure to the allergen and can range from mild to severe. If you experience severe or concerning symptoms, particularly those associated with anaphylaxis, it's important to seek immediate medical attention.

Identifying And Tracking Allergy Triggers

Identifying and tracking allergy triggers can be helpful in managing and avoiding allergic reactions. Here are some steps to identify and track allergy triggers:

Keep a Symptom Diary: Start by keeping a detailed record of your allergy symptoms, including when they occur, their severity, and any potential triggers you suspect. Note down specific details like the time of day, location, activities, and any exposure to potential allergens.

Pay Attention to Patterns: Look for patterns or common factors among your allergy symptoms. For example, if you consistently experience symptoms after being around pets or during a certain season, it may indicate an allergy to pet dander or seasonal allergies.

Consult an Allergist: If you're having trouble identifying your allergy triggers, consider consulting an allergist. They can perform tests, such as skin prick tests or blood tests, to help determine specific allergens that may be causing your symptoms.

Allergen Elimination: Once you have identified potential triggers, try eliminating them from your environment or routine to see if your symptoms improve. For example, if you suspect a food allergy, eliminate that food from your diet and observe any changes in symptoms.

Allergen Testing: In some cases, allergen testing may be necessary to confirm specific triggers. Allergen testing can involve exposure to small amounts of potential allergens under controlled conditions to observe any allergic reactions.

Use Allergy Tracking Apps or Tools: There are various apps and online tools available that can help you track your allergy symptoms, triggers, and medications. These tools often provide features like symptom logs, trigger identification, and reminders for taking medications.

By identifying and tracking your allergy triggers, you can make informed decisions about avoiding exposure to allergens and managing your allergy symptoms effectively. Remember to consult with a healthcare professional for personalized advice and guidance regarding your allergies.

Seeking Medical Diagnosis And Testing

Seeking medical diagnosis and testing is crucial for accurately identifying and managing allergies. If you suspect you have allergies, it is recommended to consult with a healthcare professional, such as an allergist or immunologist. Here are the steps typically involved in the diagnostic process:

Medical History: Your healthcare provider will begin by taking a detailed medical history, including asking about your symptoms, their duration, and any potential triggers or patterns you have noticed.

Physical Examination: A physical examination may be performed to assess any visible signs of allergic reactions, such as skin rashes or nasal congestion.

Allergy Testing: Allergy testing helps identify specific allergens that may be causing your symptoms. There are two common types of allergy tests:

Skin Prick Test: This involves applying small amounts of suspected allergens to your skin, usually on your forearm or back, and then lightly pricking or scratching the skin. If you are allergic to a particular substance, you may develop a small raised bump or redness at the test site.

Blood Test: A blood test, such as the specific IgE blood test, measures the levels of allergen-specific antibodies in your blood. This test can help determine if you have an immune response to specific allergens.

Challenge Tests: In some cases, your healthcare provider may recommend a challenge test. This involves controlled exposure to a suspected allergen to confirm or rule out an allergy. Challenge tests are typically conducted under medical supervision to monitor any allergic reactions.

Evaluation of Results: After the tests are completed, your healthcare provider will evaluate the results in the context of your symptoms and medical history to make an accurate diagnosis.

It's important to note that allergy testing should be conducted by qualified healthcare professionals to ensure accurate and safe results. They will interpret the test results, provide a diagnosis, and recommend appropriate treatment options based on your specific situation.

Remember, seeking medical diagnosis and testing is essential for managing allergies effectively. A healthcare professional can provide personalized advice, develop an appropriate treatment plan, and help you understand your specific allergies and triggers.

III. Managing Allergies through Lifestyle Changes

Allergen Avoidance Strategies

Allergen avoidance strategies are important for managing allergies and reducing the frequency and severity of allergic reactions. Here are some common allergen avoidance strategies:

Identify and Avoid Triggers: Determine the specific allergens that trigger your allergies. This can be done through medical diagnosis and testing. Once identified, take steps to avoid or minimize exposure to these allergens.

Pollen Allergies:

- Check pollen forecasts and stay indoors when pollen

levels are high.

- Keep windows closed during peak pollen seasons.
- Use air purifiers with HEPA filters in your home.
- Remove clothes and shower after spending time outdoors.

Dust Mite Allergies:

- Use dust mite-proof mattress and pillow covers.
- Wash bedding regularly in hot water.
- Vacuum and dust your home frequently.
- Reduce clutter to minimize dust accumulation.

Pet Allergies:

- Keep pets out of bedrooms and other areas where you spend a lot of time.
- Wash your hands after touching pets.
- Vacuum and clean your home regularly to remove pet dander.
- Consider hypoallergenic pet breeds or alternative pets that are less likely to trigger allergies.

Mold Allergies:

- Control humidity levels in your home to prevent mold growth.
- Use dehumidifiers in damp areas, such as basements.
- Fix any water leaks or moisture issues promptly.
- Clean and dry areas prone to mold, such as bathrooms, regularly.

Food Allergies:

- Read food labels carefully and avoid foods that contain allergens you are sensitive to.
- Inform restaurants and food establishments about your food allergies.
- Prepare and cook your own meals to have better control over ingredients.
- Be cautious of cross-contamination in shared cooking

and dining spaces.

Insect Sting Allergies:

- Wear protective clothing, such as long sleeves and pants, when outdoors.
- Avoid wearing bright-colored or floral-patterned clothing that may attract insects.
- Use insect repellents when spending time outdoors.
- Be cautious around areas where insects are likely to be present, such as gardens or garbage bins.

Remember, allergen avoidance strategies may vary depending on the specific allergens you are allergic to. It's important to work closely with your healthcare provider or allergist to develop a personalized plan and receive guidance on allergen avoidance techniques specific to your allergies.

Creating An Allergy-Friendly Home Environment

Creating an allergy-friendly home environment is essential for individuals with allergies to minimize their exposure to allergens and reduce symptoms. Here are some tips to create an allergy-friendly home:

Keep it Clean:

- Regularly clean your home to remove dust, pet dander, and other allergens.
- Vacuum carpets and rugs using a vacuum cleaner with a HEPA filter.
- Dust surfaces with a damp cloth to prevent allergens from becoming airborne.
- Wash bedding, curtains, and soft furnishings regularly in hot water to remove allergens.
- Use allergen-proof covers for mattresses, pillows, and comforters.

Maintain Optimal Humidity Levels:

- Keep humidity levels in your home between 30-50% to prevent mold and dust mite growth.
- Use dehumidifiers in damp areas like basements or bathrooms.
- Fix any water leaks or plumbing issues promptly to prevent moisture buildup.

Remove Allergen Traps:

- Remove or minimize items that can accumulate dust, such as stuffed animals, heavy curtains, and excessive decorations.
- Opt for blinds or washable curtains instead of heavy drapes.
- Declutter your home to reduce dust and allergen accumulation.

Control Pet Allergens:

- If you have pet allergies, consider keeping pets out of certain areas, especially bedrooms.
- Vacuum and clean your home regularly to remove pet dander.
- Bathe pets frequently to reduce allergens on their fur.
- Use a HEPA air purifier to help capture pet allergens.

Improve Indoor Air Quality:

- Open windows when outdoor pollen levels are low to improve ventilation.
- Use air purifiers with HEPA filters to remove airborne allergens.
- Avoid smoking or exposure to secondhand smoke in the home.

Be Mindful of Cleaning Products:

- Choose hypoallergenic, fragrance-free, and non-toxic cleaning products.
- Avoid using products that can trigger allergies or sensitivities.
- Opt for natural alternatives like vinegar and baking soda for cleaning.

Regularly Maintain HVAC Systems:

- Clean or replace air filters in heating, ventilation, and air conditioning (HVAC) systems regularly.
- Consider using high-efficiency filters to trap more allergens.
- Schedule regular professional maintenance of your HVAC system to keep it clean and efficient.

Remember, every individual's allergies may differ, so it's important to identify specific triggers and work with your healthcare provider or allergist to develop a customized plan for creating an allergy-friendly home environment.

Tips For Managing Allergies At Work And In Public Spaces

Managing allergies at work and in public spaces can be challenging, but with some proactive measures, you can minimize exposure to allergens and reduce symptoms. Here are some tips for managing allergies in these environments:

Communicate with Others:

- Inform your colleagues and supervisor about your allergies so they can be considerate and help create an allergy-friendly workspace.
- Request to have your workspace away from potential allergen sources like dusty areas, strong scents, or pet dander.

Keep Your Workspace Clean:

- Regularly clean your desk and surrounding area to remove dust and allergens.
- Use a damp cloth to wipe surfaces instead of dry dusting, as dry dusting can stir up allergens into the air.
- Consider using a desk air purifier with a HEPA filter to help remove airborne allergens.

Avoid Food Allergens:

- If you have food allergies, be cautious about eating in common areas or sharing utensils.
- Read food labels carefully and be aware of potential cross-contamination in shared spaces like refrigerators or microwaves.

Manage Air Quality:

- If possible, keep windows closed to prevent outdoor allergens from entering the workspace.
- If air quality is a concern, consider using a personal air purifier or wearing a mask designed to filter allergens.

Be Mindful of Scents:

- Avoid wearing strong perfumes, colognes, or scented lotions that may trigger allergies in others.
- Politely request colleagues to refrain from using strong fragrances in the workspace.

Plan for Outdoor Allergens:

- Check pollen forecasts and plan your outdoor breaks accordingly.
- Consider wearing sunglasses and a hat to protect your eyes and face from allergens.
- Change your clothes and wash your hands after spending time outdoors to remove pollen.

Carry Medications:

- Keep your allergy medications, such as antihistamines or epinephrine auto-injectors (if prescribed), easily accessible at work.
- If necessary, inform your colleagues or supervisor about your emergency action plan for severe allergic reactions.

Advocate for Accommodations:

- If your allergies significantly impact your work, discuss possible accommodations with your supervisor or HR department.
- This may include adjustments to your workspace, flexible scheduling to avoid peak allergy times, or remote work options.

Remember to consult with your healthcare provider or allergist for personalized advice and strategies to manage your specific allergies in work and public settings.

Allergy-Friendly Travel Tips

Traveling with allergies requires some extra planning and precautions to ensure a safe and enjoyable trip. Here are some allergy-friendly travel tips:

Research Your Destination:

- Before you travel, research the allergens commonly found in your destination. This includes food allergies, pollen levels, air quality, and any other relevant allergens.
- Find out if there are any local customs or specific foods that may contain your allergens.

Pack Allergy Medications and Supplies:

- Bring an ample supply of your allergy medications, including antihistamines, epinephrine auto-injectors (if needed), and any other prescribed medications.
- Carry your medications with you in your carry-on luggage or purse, rather than checking them in.

Notify Your Travel Companions:

- If you're traveling with others, inform them about your allergies and provide them with instructions on how to respond in case of an allergic reaction.
- Ensure they know how to use an epinephrine auto-injector if you have severe allergies.

Plan Your Meals:

- If you have food allergies, research restaurants and local cuisine options that cater to dietary restrictions.
- Communicate your food allergies to restaurant staff and ask about the ingredients and preparation methods.
- Consider packing some safe snacks or meals for times when allergen-free options may be limited.

Read Labels and Pack Snacks:

- Pack allergen-free snacks and foods that you know are safe for you to eat, especially for long flights or road trips.
- Read labels carefully when purchasing snacks or meals during your travel to avoid any potential allergens.

Communicate with Airlines and Hotels:

- If you have severe allergies, inform the airline in advance about your condition and any specific accommodations you may require.
- Contact hotels or accommodations to inquire about allergen-free rooms or rooms with hypoallergenic bedding.

Carry Allergy Alert Cards:

- Consider carrying allergy alert cards or a medical ID bracelet that clearly states your allergies and emergency contact information.
- These cards can be useful in case of an allergic reaction or if you need to communicate your allergies in a foreign language.

Be Prepared for Allergic Reactions:

- Familiarize yourself with emergency numbers and healthcare facilities at your destination.
- Research local hospitals or clinics that can provide medical assistance in case of an allergic reaction.

Remember to consult with your allergist or healthcare provider for personalized advice and recommendations based on your specific allergies before you travel. They can provide you with additional tips and precautions based on your individual needs.

IV. Natural Remedies for Allergy Relief

Herbal Remedies And Supplements

Herbal remedies and supplements are often used as complementary approaches to support health and well-being. While they may offer potential benefits, it's important to use them with caution and under the guidance of a healthcare professional, especially if you have allergies or medical conditions. Here are some common herbal remedies and supplements that are believed to have potential benefits:

Butterbur: Butterbur is a herb that has been used traditionally for allergies, particularly seasonal allergies. It may help reduce symptoms such as sneezing, nasal congestion, and itchy eyes.

Quercetin: Quercetin is a flavonoid found in many fruits and vegetables. It has antioxidant and anti-inflammatory properties and is believed to help stabilize mast cells, which release histamine during allergic reactions.

Stinging Nettle: Stinging nettle is often used to alleviate symptoms of allergies, particularly hay fever. It may help reduce inflammation and ease symptoms like sneezing and itching.

Probiotics: Probiotics are beneficial bacteria that support gut health. Some research suggests that certain strains of probiotics may help modulate the immune system and reduce the severity of allergic reactions.

Vitamin C: Vitamin C is an antioxidant that may have anti-allergic properties. It is believed to help reduce the release of histamine and alleviate symptoms like nasal congestion and sneezing.

Omega-3 Fatty Acids: Omega-3 fatty acids, commonly found in fish oil supplements, have anti-inflammatory properties and may help reduce inflammation associated with allergies.

Bromelain: Bromelain is an enzyme found in pineapple stems. It may have anti-inflammatory properties and could potentially help reduce nasal congestion and sinus inflammation.

It's important to note that while some people may find relief from these herbal remedies and supplements, scientific evidence supporting their effectiveness for allergies is often limited and inconsistent. Additionally, they can interact with medications or cause adverse effects in certain individuals. It's advisable to consult with a healthcare professional or an integrative medicine practitioner before starting any herbal remedies or supplements, especially if you have allergies or any underlying health conditions. They can assess your individual situation and provide guidance on appropriate and safe usage.

Nasal Rinses And Saline Sprays

Nasal rinses and saline sprays are commonly used as natural remedies to alleviate symptoms of allergies, sinus congestion, and nasal irritation. They work by flushing out irritants, allergens, and excess mucus from the nasal passages, helping to relieve congestion and improve breathing. Here are some key points about nasal rinses and saline sprays:

Neti Pot: A neti pot is a small vessel used to pour a saline solution into one nostril, allowing it to flow through the nasal passages and out the other nostril. It helps clear the nasal passages, reduce congestion, and remove irritants and allergens.

Saline Nasal Sprays: Saline nasal sprays contain a saltwater solution that can be sprayed directly into the nostrils. They provide moisture to dry nasal passages and help rinse away mucus, irritants, and allergens.

Benefits: Nasal rinses and saline sprays can provide temporary relief from nasal congestion, sinus pressure, and nasal irritation caused by allergies or other nasal conditions. They can help soothe dry nasal passages, reduce inflammation, and improve breathing.

Usage: Follow the instructions provided with the specific product you are using. Typically, a saline solution is mixed with lukewarm distilled or sterile water for use with a neti pot. Saline nasal sprays can be used multiple times a day, as needed, to keep the nasal passages moist and clear.

Safety Precautions: It's essential to use sterile water or distilled water when preparing the saline solution to avoid introducing harmful bacteria into the nasal passages. It's also important to clean and properly maintain the neti pot or nasal spray bottle to prevent bacterial growth.

Side Effects: Nasal rinses and saline sprays are generally safe when used correctly. However, improper usage or using non-sterile water can lead to infections. Some individuals may experience temporary mild discomfort, such as a slight burning or stinging sensation, which typically subsides quickly.

Consultation: If you have any underlying nasal conditions or concerns, it's best to consult with a healthcare professional before using nasal rinses or saline sprays to ensure they are appropriate for your specific situation.

Nasal rinses and saline sprays can be effective in providing temporary relief and promoting nasal health. However, if you have persistent or severe nasal symptoms, it's important to consult with a healthcare professional for a proper evaluation and guidance on appropriate treatment options.

Breathing Exercises And Relaxation Techniques

Breathing exercises and relaxation techniques can be helpful tools for managing stress, promoting relaxation, and improving overall well-being. They can also be beneficial in alleviating symptoms related to allergies, such as respiratory congestion and difficulty breathing. Here are some common breathing exercises and relaxation techniques:

Deep Breathing: Deep breathing involves taking slow, deep breaths, filling the lungs fully with air, and then exhaling slowly. This technique helps activate the body's relaxation response and promotes a sense of calm.

Diaphragmatic Breathing: Also known as belly breathing, diaphragmatic breathing involves breathing deeply into the abdomen, allowing the diaphragm to fully expand. This technique helps promote relaxation, reduce stress, and improve oxygenation.

Alternate Nostril Breathing: This technique involves breathing through one nostril at a time while closing off the other nostril with the fingers. It helps balance the flow of energy in the body, promotes relaxation, and enhances mental clarity.

Box Breathing: Box breathing involves inhaling slowly for a specific count, holding the breath for the same count, exhaling slowly for the count, and then holding the breath again for the count. This technique helps calm the mind, reduce anxiety, and improve focus.

Progressive Muscle Relaxation: This technique involves systematically tensing and relaxing different muscle groups in the body, promoting relaxation and releasing tension.

Guided Imagery: Guided imagery involves visualizing calming and peaceful scenes or experiences to promote relaxation and reduce stress.

Mindfulness Meditation: Mindfulness meditation involves focusing attention on the present moment, observing thoughts and sensations without judgment. This practice promotes relaxation, reduces stress, and enhances overall well-being.

Yoga and Tai Chi: These mind-body practices combine movement, breath control, and mindfulness to promote relaxation, flexibility, and overall physical and mental well-being.

When practicing breathing exercises and relaxation techniques, find a quiet and comfortable space where you can fully focus and relax. Start with a few minutes each day and gradually increase the duration as you become more comfortable. Regular practice can help build resilience to stress, improve respiratory function, and enhance overall relaxation and well-being.

Essential Oils For Allergy Relief

While some essential oils may offer relief from allergy symptoms, it's important to note that individual responses can vary. It's recommended to consult with a healthcare professional or aromatherapist before using essential oils for allergy relief. Here are a few essential oils that are commonly used:

Peppermint: Peppermint essential oil is known for its cooling and decongestant properties. It may help relieve nasal congestion and soothe respiratory discomfort.

Eucalyptus: Eucalyptus essential oil has expectorant properties and can help clear congestion and promote easier breathing.

Lavender: Lavender essential oil has calming and anti-inflammatory properties. It may help reduce inflammation and provide relaxation during allergic reactions.

Lemon: Lemon essential oil is often used for its cleansing properties. It may help support the immune system and promote a healthy respiratory system.

Tea Tree: Tea tree essential oil has antimicrobial and anti-inflammatory properties. It may help alleviate respiratory symptoms and support the immune system.

It's important to dilute essential oils properly before use and perform a patch test to check for any allergic reactions. Essential oils can be diffused, diluted and applied topically, or added to bathwater for inhalation. Remember to use them in moderation and discontinue use if any adverse reactions occur.

V. Medical Treatments for Allergies

Over-The-Counter Medications For Symptom Relief

There are several over-the-counter medications available that can provide relief from allergy symptoms. These medications can help alleviate symptoms such as nasal congestion, sneezing, itching, and watery eyes. It's important to read and follow the instructions on the packaging and consult with a healthcare professional if you have any questions or concerns. Here are some common types of over-the-counter allergy medications:

Antihistamines: These medications block the effects of histamine, a substance released during an allergic reaction. They can help relieve symptoms like itching, sneezing, and runny nose. Some examples include loratadine, cetirizine, and fexofenadine.

Decongestants: Decongestants help relieve nasal congestion by narrowing blood vessels in the nasal passages. They can provide temporary relief from stuffy nose symptoms. Examples include pseudoephedrine and phenylephrine. However, decongestants should be used with caution and only for short periods of time, as long-term use can lead to rebound congestion.

Nasal sprays: Nasal sprays can help reduce nasal congestion and inflammation. There are different types available, including saline sprays for moisturizing and clearing nasal passages, as well as steroid nasal sprays that can provide more significant relief from allergy symptoms.

Eye drops: Eye drops can help relieve itchy and watery eyes caused by allergies. There are antihistamine eye drops and lubricating eye drops available over the counter.

It's important to note that while these medications can provide temporary relief, they may not address the underlying cause of allergies. If symptoms persist or worsen, it's advisable to consult with a healthcare professional for further evaluation and treatment options.

Prescription Medications For Allergies

When over-the-counter medications are not sufficient in managing allergy symptoms, a healthcare professional may prescribe stronger medications. These prescription medications are typically recommended for individuals with more severe or persistent allergy symptoms. Here are some common types of prescription medications used for allergies:

Prescription Antihistamines: These are stronger versions of over-the-counter antihistamines and can provide more effective relief for allergy symptoms such as itching, sneezing, and runny nose.

Prescription Nasal Sprays: There are different types of prescription nasal sprays available, including corticosteroid nasal sprays that help reduce inflammation and congestion in the nasal passages. They can provide significant relief for nasal symptoms.

Leukotriene Modifiers: These medications work by blocking the effects of certain chemicals in the body that contribute to allergic reactions. They can be helpful in managing symptoms like congestion, wheezing, and coughing.

Immunotherapy: In cases of severe allergies or when other treatments are not effective, immunotherapy may be recommended. This involves regular injections or sublingual tablets that expose the body to small amounts of allergens over time, helping the immune system develop tolerance and reducing the severity of allergic reactions.

It's important to consult with a healthcare professional to determine the most appropriate prescription medication based on your specific allergy symptoms and medical history. They can assess your condition and provide personalized recommendations for effective management of your allergies.

Allergy Shots (Immunotherapy)

Allergy shots, also known as immunotherapy, are a treatment option for individuals with severe allergies or allergies that do not respond well to other treatments. Here's some information about allergy shots:

How it works: Allergy shots work by gradually exposing the body to small amounts of allergens, such as pollen, pet dander, or dust mites, over a period of time. The injections contain extracts of specific allergens to which the person is allergic. The doses are increased gradually to help the immune system develop tolerance to these allergens.

Benefits: The primary goal of allergy shots is to reduce the severity of allergic reactions over time. They can help alleviate symptoms such as nasal congestion, sneezing, itching, and wheezing. Allergy shots can also provide long-term relief and potentially reduce the need for other medications.

Treatment duration: Allergy shots involve a series of injections given on a regular schedule, typically starting with a buildup phase and transitioning to a maintenance phase. The buildup phase involves more frequent injections, usually one to two times a week. Once the maintenance dose is reached, the injections are given less frequently, usually every few weeks or months. The duration of treatment varies, but it typically lasts for several years.

Effectiveness: Allergy shots have been shown to be effective in reducing allergy symptoms and the need for medication in many individuals. However, the degree of improvement can vary from person to person. It may take several months to a year or more of consistent treatment to notice significant results.

Safety considerations: Allergy shots are generally safe, but there is a potential risk of allergic reactions to the injections. These reactions are usually mild and can include redness, swelling, or itching at the injection site. In rare cases, more serious reactions such as anaphylaxis can occur. That's why allergy shots are administered in a healthcare setting where medical professionals can monitor for any adverse reactions.

Allergy shots are typically prescribed and administered by allergists or immunologists. If you are considering allergy shots as a treatment option, it's important to consult with a healthcare professional who specializes in allergies to determine if this approach is suitable for you. They can assess your specific allergy triggers and symptoms, and create a personalized treatment plan to help manage your allergies effectively.

Alternative Treatments (Acupuncture, Chiropractic Care, Etc.)

Alternative treatments can be considered as complementary approaches to managing allergies. While they may not directly target the underlying immune response like medications or immunotherapy, some individuals find relief and symptom management through these practices. Here are a few alternative treatments that are sometimes used for allergies:

Acupuncture: Acupuncture is an ancient Chinese practice that involves inserting thin needles into specific points on the body. It is believed to help balance the body's energy flow and stimulate natural healing. Some individuals with allergies have reported improvement in symptoms such as congestion, sneezing, and itching after acupuncture sessions.

Chiropractic care: Chiropractic care focuses on the alignment of the spine and the proper functioning of the nervous system. Some chiropractors may use spinal adjustments and other techniques to help improve the body's overall function, including the immune system. While there is limited scientific evidence specifically linking chiropractic care to allergy relief, some individuals have reported positive results.

Herbal remedies: Certain herbs and natural supplements have been traditionally used to alleviate allergy symptoms. Examples include butterbur, stinging nettle, quercetin, and bromelain. However, it's important to note that the effectiveness and safety of herbal remedies can vary, and it's advisable to consult with a healthcare professional before trying any new supplements.

Nasal irrigation: Nasal irrigation, also known as nasal rinsing or nasal douching, involves using a saline solution to flush out the nasal passages. This practice can help remove allergens, reduce congestion, and alleviate symptoms. Neti pots, squeeze bottles, or nasal sprays can be used for nasal irrigation.

It's crucial to approach alternative treatments with caution and consult with qualified healthcare professionals. They can provide guidance based on your individual needs, medical history, and allergies. It's also important to remember that alternative treatments should not replace evidence-based medical treatments for severe allergies or anaphylaxis. It's always a good idea to discuss any alternative treatment options with your healthcare provider to ensure they are safe and suitable for your specific situation.

VI. Managing Allergies in Specific Scenarios

Allergies In Children And Infants

Allergies can affect children and infants just as they can affect adults. In fact, allergies often develop during childhood. Here are some important points to consider about allergies in children and infants:

Common allergens: The most common allergens in children include food allergens (such as cow's milk, eggs, peanuts, tree nuts, wheat, soy, fish, and shellfish), environmental allergens (such as pollen, dust mites, pet dander, and mold), and insect venom. It's also possible for children to develop allergies to medications or latex.

Symptoms: Allergic reactions in children can manifest in various ways, depending on the type of allergy. Food allergies may cause digestive issues (e.g., vomiting, diarrhea), skin rashes, swelling, difficulty breathing, or anaphylaxis (a severe and potentially life-threatening reaction). Environmental allergies can lead to nasal congestion, sneezing, itchy and watery eyes, coughing, wheezing, and skin reactions (e.g., eczema).

Diagnosis: If you suspect that your child has allergies, it's important to consult with a pediatrician or allergist. They will evaluate your child's symptoms, medical history, and may recommend allergy testing. Common tests include skin prick tests, blood tests (such as IgE-specific antibody tests), and oral food challenges for suspected food allergies.

Management and treatment: Allergy management in children often involves a combination of allergen avoidance, medications, and, in some cases, immunotherapy. For food allergies, strict avoidance of the allergenic food is necessary. Environmental allergies can be managed through allergen avoidance strategies, such as using allergen-proof bedding, keeping indoor spaces clean, and minimizing exposure to known triggers. Medications such as antihistamines, nasal sprays, and asthma inhalers may be prescribed to alleviate symptoms. In certain cases, allergen immunotherapy (allergy shots) may be recommended to desensitize the child's immune system to specific allergens.

Education and awareness: It's important for parents, caregivers, teachers, and other individuals involved in a child's care to be educated about their allergies. This includes recognizing symptoms of an allergic reaction, understanding the child's specific triggers and management strategies, and knowing how to respond in case of an emergency. Allergy action plans and carrying necessary medications (e.g., epinephrine auto-injectors) should be part of the child's care plan.

If you suspect your child has allergies, it's best to consult with a healthcare professional who specializes in pediatric allergies. They can provide proper diagnosis, guidance, and an individualized treatment plan for your child's specific needs.

Allergies During Pregnancy

Allergies during pregnancy can present unique challenges for expectant mothers. Here are some important points to consider about allergies during pregnancy:

Hormonal changes: Pregnancy causes various hormonal changes in the body, which can affect the immune system. These changes may lead to new allergies or exacerbate existing ones. Some pregnant women may experience relief from their allergies during pregnancy, while others may experience an increase in symptoms.

Common allergens: The same allergens that cause allergies in non-pregnant individuals can trigger allergic reactions in pregnant women as well. Common allergens include pollen, dust mites, pet dander, mold, certain foods, and insect venom.

Medications and treatments: When managing allergies during pregnancy, it's important to consider the potential risks and benefits of medications and treatments. Some allergy medications, especially oral antihistamines and decongestants, may not be recommended during pregnancy due to potential risks to the developing fetus. However, some topical nasal sprays, saline rinses, and certain antihistamines may be considered safe for use during pregnancy. It's crucial to consult with a healthcare professional, such as an obstetrician or allergist, to discuss the safest options for managing allergies while pregnant.

Allergen avoidance: Whenever possible, allergen avoidance is a key strategy for managing allergies during pregnancy. This may involve reducing exposure to known allergens, such as keeping indoor spaces clean, using allergen-proof bedding, avoiding certain foods or ingredients, and minimizing exposure to environmental triggers like pollen or pet dander.

Consultation with healthcare professionals: If you have allergies and are pregnant or planning to become pregnant, it's important to consult with your healthcare provider. They can provide guidance on managing your allergies during pregnancy, suggest safe treatment options, and help you navigate any potential risks or concerns.

Allergy testing: In some cases, allergy testing may be recommended during pregnancy if it's necessary to identify specific allergens causing severe symptoms or if it's important for treatment decisions. The timing and type of allergy testing will be determined by your healthcare provider, taking into consideration the potential risks and benefits.

It's important to prioritize your health and well-being during pregnancy, including the management of your allergies. By working closely with your healthcare provider, you can develop an individualized plan that minimizes risks and ensures the best possible care for you and your baby.

Allergies And Aging

As individuals age, there can be changes in the immune system and the body's response to allergens. Here are some important points to consider regarding allergies and aging:

Increased sensitivity: Older adults may develop increased sensitivity to certain allergens or experience allergies for the first time later in life. This can be attributed to changes in the immune system and a decreased ability to tolerate allergens.

Changes in symptoms: Allergy symptoms in older adults may manifest differently compared to younger individuals. For example, nasal congestion and post-nasal drip may be more prominent, while classic symptoms like sneezing and itchy eyes may be less pronounced.

Co-existing health conditions: Older adults often have other health conditions that can complicate allergy management. Conditions such as asthma, chronic obstructive pulmonary disease (COPD), or cardiovascular disease can interact with allergies and exacerbate symptoms.

Medications and interactions: Older adults may be taking multiple medications for various health conditions. It's important to be aware of potential interactions between allergy medications and other medications, as well as any contraindications for certain medications in individuals with specific health conditions.

Delayed diagnosis: Allergies in older adults may be underdiagnosed or misdiagnosed due to the overlap of symptoms with other health conditions. It's important for older adults to communicate their symptoms clearly to healthcare providers and seek proper evaluation if they suspect allergies.

Management strategies: Allergen avoidance remains an important strategy for managing allergies in older adults. This may involve reducing exposure to common allergens in the home, maintaining clean indoor air quality, and taking precautions when spending time outdoors during high pollen seasons. Medications, such as antihistamines, nasal sprays, or eye drops, may be prescribed to alleviate symptoms, but the choice of medication should be made in consultation with a healthcare provider, taking into consideration any existing health conditions or medication interactions.

It's important for older adults to work closely with their healthcare providers, including allergists or immunologists, to manage their allergies effectively. Regular communication, medication reviews, and tailored treatment plans can help ensure that allergies are properly diagnosed and managed in the context of an individual's overall health and well-being.

Allergies And Comorbid Conditions (Asthma, Eczema, Etc.)

Allergies can often coexist with other conditions, such as asthma, eczema, and sinusitis. Here's some information about the relationship between allergies and these comorbid conditions:

Asthma: Allergies and asthma often go hand in hand. Allergic triggers, such as pollen, dust mites, pet dander, or mold, can provoke asthma symptoms in individuals with allergic asthma. These symptoms may include wheezing, shortness of breath, coughing, and chest tightness. Managing both allergies and asthma is crucial to control symptoms and prevent exacerbations. In some cases, allergy testing and specific allergen immunotherapy (allergy shots) may be recommended to help reduce asthma symptoms triggered by allergens.

Eczema (Atopic Dermatitis): Eczema is a chronic skin condition characterized by dry, itchy, and inflamed skin. Allergies, particularly food allergies and environmental allergens, can trigger or worsen eczema symptoms in some individuals. This is known as atopic dermatitis. Identifying and avoiding allergens that trigger eczema flare-ups, such as certain foods or irritants, can be helpful in managing the condition. Additionally, topical treatments, moisturizers, and medications prescribed by a dermatologist can help control eczema symptoms.

Sinusitis: Allergies can contribute to the development or exacerbation of sinusitis, which is the inflammation of the sinuses. When allergens such as pollen or dust mites are inhaled, they can trigger an allergic reaction in the nasal passages and sinuses, leading to inflammation and blockage. This can result in symptoms such as nasal congestion, facial pain or pressure, post-nasal drip, and sinus headaches. Managing allergies through allergen avoidance, medications, and nasal irrigation can help reduce the frequency and severity of sinusitis episodes.

Allergic Rhinitis: Allergic rhinitis, also known as hay fever, is an allergic response that primarily affects the nose and eyes. It is characterized by symptoms such as sneezing, runny or stuffy nose, itchy and watery eyes, and itching of the throat or ears. Allergic rhinitis can occur on its own or coexist with other conditions like asthma and eczema. Treatment options for allergic rhinitis include allergen avoidance, over-the-counter or prescription medications (antihistamines, nasal sprays), and immunotherapy for severe or persistent cases.

Managing allergies and their comorbid conditions often involves a comprehensive approach. This may include identifying and avoiding allergens, using medications to control symptoms, and working closely with healthcare providers, such as allergists, pulmonologists, dermatologists, or otolaryngologists, to develop personalized treatment plans. Regular follow-ups and communication with healthcare providers are important for ongoing management and optimal control of both allergies and comorbid conditions.

VII. Allergy Prevention and Long-Term Management

Strategies For Preventing Allergies

While it's not always possible to prevent allergies entirely, there are several strategies you can adopt to reduce your exposure to allergens and minimize the risk of developing allergies. Here are some prevention strategies:

Identify and avoid allergens: If you know you're allergic to certain substances, such as pollen, dust mites, pet dander, or certain foods, take steps to minimize your exposure. This may involve keeping windows closed during high pollen seasons, using dust mite-proof covers for bedding, keeping pets out of bedrooms, and avoiding specific foods or ingredients.

Keep indoor air clean: Improve indoor air quality by using air purifiers with HEPA filters, regularly cleaning and vacuuming your home, and minimizing the use of carpets and upholstered furniture that can trap allergens. Consider using hypoallergenic bedding and washing it frequently in hot water to remove allergens.

Control humidity levels: High humidity can promote the growth of mold and dust mites, which are common allergens. Use dehumidifiers in damp areas of your home, such as basements, bathrooms, and laundry rooms. Keep humidity levels between 30% and 50% to prevent the proliferation of allergens.

Practice good hygiene: Wash your hands regularly, especially after being outside or coming into contact with potential allergens. This can help prevent allergens from spreading and reduce your risk of exposure.

Be cautious with pets: If you're allergic to pet dander, consider avoiding pets that trigger your allergies. If you have pets, bathe them regularly and keep them out of bedrooms and other areas where you spend a lot of time.

Take precautions during outdoor activities: When outdoor allergens, such as pollen, are high, limit your time outdoors, especially on windy days. Check pollen forecasts and plan outdoor activities accordingly. After spending time outside, change your clothes, wash your face, and rinse your hair to remove allergens.

Consider allergen immunotherapy: Allergen immunotherapy, commonly known as allergy shots, may be recommended for individuals with severe allergies. This treatment involves regular injections of small amounts of allergens to desensitize the immune system and reduce allergic reactions. Consult with an allergist to determine if this treatment is appropriate for you.

It's important to note that these strategies may not guarantee the prevention of allergies, especially if you have a genetic predisposition or are already sensitized to certain allergens. If you suspect you have allergies or are at risk, consult with an allergist who can provide personalized guidance and recommend appropriate preventive measures based on your specific situation.

Creating An Allergy Action Plan

Creating an allergy action plan is an important step in managing and responding to allergies effectively. An allergy action plan is a personalized document that outlines the specific actions to take in the event of an allergic reaction. Here are some steps to create an allergy action plan:

Consult with an allergist: Work closely with an allergist or healthcare provider to develop an allergy action plan. They will assess your specific allergies, triggers, and symptoms, and provide guidance on appropriate actions.

Understand your symptoms: Be aware of the typical symptoms you experience during an allergic reaction. Common symptoms include itching, hives, swelling, nasal congestion, sneezing, wheezing, coughing, and difficulty breathing. Note any severe symptoms that may require immediate medical attention.

Identify triggers: Determine the specific allergens that trigger your allergic reactions, such as certain foods, medications, insect stings, or environmental factors like pollen or pet dander. Understanding your triggers is crucial for prevention and response.

Know your medications: Discuss with your healthcare provider the appropriate medications to have on hand for allergy management. This may include antihistamines for mild symptoms and epinephrine auto-injectors (e.g., EpiPen) for severe allergic reactions (anaphylaxis). Understand how and when to use these medications.

Communicate with others: Inform key people in your life about your allergies, including family members, friends, coworkers, and teachers. Make sure they understand the signs of an allergic reaction and how to respond in an emergency situation.

Develop an emergency plan: Create a clear set of instructions on what to do in case of a severe allergic reaction. Include step-by-step procedures for using an epinephrine auto-injector, when to call emergency services, and any additional emergency contacts.

Educate yourself and others: Learn about allergy triggers, prevention strategies, and the signs of an allergic reaction. Share this knowledge with those around you to create a supportive and informed network.

Carry identification: Wear a medical alert bracelet or carry a card indicating your allergies, especially if you have severe allergies or are at risk of anaphylaxis. This can help others identify your condition in case of an emergency.

Regularly review and update: Review your allergy action plan periodically to ensure it is up to date. Update any changes in triggers, medications, emergency contacts, or other relevant information.

Remember, an allergy action plan is a personalized document, so consult with your healthcare provider for specific recommendations and guidance based on your allergies and medical history. By having a well-defined action plan, you can be prepared to manage allergic reactions effectively and minimize potential risks.

Regular Check-Ups And Monitoring

Regular check-ups and monitoring are crucial for managing allergies effectively. Here's why they are important:

Evaluation of symptoms: Regular check-ups with your allergist or healthcare provider allow for ongoing evaluation of your allergy symptoms. They can assess the frequency and severity of your symptoms, identify any changes or patterns, and adjust your treatment plan accordingly.

Review of triggers: Regular monitoring helps you identify and track your allergy triggers. By discussing your daily activities, exposures, and any changes in your environment, your healthcare provider can help you pinpoint potential triggers and develop strategies for avoidance.

Medication management: Check-ups provide an opportunity to review your current medications, including prescription and over-the-counter allergy medications. Your healthcare provider can assess their effectiveness, discuss any side effects or concerns, and make necessary adjustments to your treatment regimen.

Preventive measures: Regular check-ups allow for discussions about preventive measures to minimize exposure to allergens. For example, your healthcare provider can advise you on strategies for reducing exposure to pollen during allergy season or implementing allergen control measures in your home.

Allergy testing: If needed, regular check-ups may include allergy testing to determine specific allergens that trigger your symptoms. Testing can help identify additional allergies that may have developed over time or confirm suspected triggers. This information is valuable for developing an effective treatment plan.

Asthma management: If you have allergies and asthma, regular check-ups are particularly important. Your healthcare provider can monitor your lung function, assess asthma control, and make necessary adjustments to your asthma management plan. This can help prevent asthma exacerbations triggered by allergies.

Education and support: Regular check-ups provide an opportunity for education and support. You can discuss any concerns, ask questions, and receive guidance on managing your allergies effectively. Your healthcare provider can provide updates on the latest treatments and research in the field of allergy management.

Remember to keep a record of your symptoms, triggers, and any changes in your condition between check-ups. This information will be helpful during your appointments and ensure comprehensive and accurate discussions with your healthcare provider.

Overall, regular check-ups and monitoring play a vital role in managing allergies. They help ensure that your treatment plan is optimized, provide opportunities for preventive measures, and support your overall well-being. Schedule regular appointments with your allergist or healthcare provider to stay on top of your allergy management and maintain a healthy and comfortable lifestyle.

Allergy Support Groups And Resources

Participating in allergy support groups and accessing relevant resources can provide valuable information, education, and emotional support for individuals and families dealing with allergies. Here are some options to consider:

Allergy Support Groups: Joining local or online support groups specifically focused on allergies can connect you with others who share similar experiences. These groups often provide a platform for sharing stories, tips, and advice, as well as emotional support. You can search for local support groups through community centers, hospitals, or allergy clinics, or explore online communities and forums dedicated to allergies.

Allergy Organizations and Associations: Numerous organizations and associations are dedicated to providing resources and support for individuals with allergies. Examples include:

Allergy & Asthma Network: A nonprofit organization that provides educational resources, support, and advocacy for individuals with allergies and asthma.

Asthma and Allergy Foundation of America (AAFA): An organization that offers educational resources, support networks, and advocacy for individuals with allergies and asthma.

Food Allergy Research & Education (FARE): A nonprofit organization focused on food allergy awareness, education, and support for individuals and families.

American Academy of Allergy, Asthma & Immunology (AAAAI): A professional organization that offers patient resources and information on allergies, asthma, and immunology.

Allergy Websites and Online Resources: Several websites provide comprehensive information, tips, and resources related to allergies. Some reputable sources include:

Mayo Clinic: The Mayo Clinic website offers reliable information on various allergies, symptoms, causes, treatments, and prevention strategies.

American College of Allergy, Asthma & Immunology (ACAAI): The ACAAI website provides patient resources, educational materials, and tools for managing allergies and related conditions.

National Institute of Allergy and Infectious Diseases (NIAID): NIAID offers allergy-related research updates, educational resources, and information on clinical trials.

Allergy Apps: There are mobile applications available that offer allergy management tools, symptom trackers, and resources. Some popular allergy apps include AllergyEats, AllergyPal, and My Pollen Forecast.

Allergist or Immunologist: Consulting with an allergist or immunologist is an important step in managing allergies. These healthcare professionals can provide personalized guidance, conduct allergy testing, and recommend appropriate treatments. They may also be aware of local support groups or resources that can be beneficial.

Remember to always verify the credibility and accuracy of the information and resources you access. Consult with your healthcare provider or allergist for specific advice and recommendations tailored to your individual needs.

By engaging with allergy support groups and accessing reliable resources, you can enhance your knowledge, find emotional support, and discover strategies for managing allergies effectively.

VIII. Dealing with Allergy Challenges and Emotional Well-being

Coping With The Emotional Impact Of Allergies

Dealing with allergies can have an emotional impact, as it can significantly affect daily life and overall well-being. Here are some strategies for coping with the emotional aspect of allergies:

Acknowledge and Validate Your Feelings: It is important to recognize and acknowledge any negative emotions or frustrations you may experience due to allergies. Understand that it is normal to feel upset, annoyed, or even discouraged at times. Validate your feelings and remind yourself that it is okay to feel the way you do.

Seek Support: Reach out to friends, family, or support groups who can provide understanding and empathy. Sharing your experiences with others who have similar allergies can offer a sense of validation and camaraderie. Online communities, forums, and social media groups focused on allergies can also be valuable sources of support.

Educate Yourself: Learn as much as you can about your

specific allergies, including triggers, symptoms, and management strategies. Understanding the condition and its impact on your life can help you feel more empowered and in control.

Communicate Effectively: Communicate your needs and concerns to your loved ones, colleagues, and healthcare professionals. Let them know how allergies affect you and what support you require. Clear and open communication can foster understanding and empathy from those around you.

Practice Self-Care: Engage in self-care activities to reduce stress and promote emotional well-being. This can include activities such as exercise, meditation, deep breathing, spending time in nature, pursuing hobbies, or engaging in relaxation techniques. Taking care of your mental and emotional health can help you cope better with the challenges of allergies.

Focus on the Positives: While allergies can be frustrating, try to focus on the positive aspects of your life and the things you can still enjoy. Look for alternative activities or foods that you can savor. Celebrate your achievements and small victories along the way.

Seek Professional Help: If your emotional well-being is significantly impacted by allergies and it becomes challenging to cope, consider seeking professional help. A mental health professional can provide guidance, support, and strategies to manage stress, anxiety, or depression related to allergies.

Remember that everyone's experience with allergies is unique, and it is essential to find coping mechanisms that work best for you. Be patient with yourself, practice self-compassion, and reach out for support when needed.

Overcoming Challenges In Social Situations

Overcoming challenges in social situations related to allergies can be a common concern. Here are some strategies to help you navigate social settings with allergies:

Communicate Your Allergies: Clearly communicate your allergies to the people you are socializing with, whether it's friends, family, or colleagues. Let them know about your specific triggers and the potential reactions you may experience. This will help others understand and be more considerate of your needs.

Plan Ahead: If you know you will be attending a social event where there may be allergens present, such as a restaurant or someone's home, plan ahead. Contact the venue or host in advance to discuss your allergies and any necessary accommodations. This may include checking the menu for allergens or asking if they can provide allergy-friendly options.

Bring Your Own Food: If you're unsure about the availability of allergen-free options at a social gathering, consider bringing your own food. This ensures you have safe and suitable options to enjoy without risking exposure to allergens.

Educate Others: Take the opportunity to educate those around you about allergies and their potential severity. Help others understand the importance of avoiding cross-contamination and the need for precautions when preparing or serving food.

Carry Medications: Always have your necessary allergy medications with you, such as antihistamines or epinephrine auto-injectors, in case of an allergic reaction. Inform close friends or family members about your allergies and where you keep your medications.

Stay Vigilant: Be cautious in social settings and avoid potential allergen exposure. Stay vigilant by reading food labels, asking about ingredients, and double-checking with the server or host if you have any doubts.

Have an Emergency Plan: Develop an emergency plan with your healthcare provider to handle severe allergic reactions. Understand the signs of anaphylaxis and know when and how to administer your emergency medication if necessary.

Seek Support: Consider joining support groups or online communities for individuals with allergies. Connecting with others who share similar experiences can provide a sense of understanding, advice, and encouragement.

Practice Self-Care: Prioritize self-care before and after social events. Allergy-related stress or anxiety can be managed by practicing relaxation techniques, engaging in activities you enjoy, and taking care of your overall well-being.

Remember, it's important to advocate for your needs and prioritize your health in social situations. With proper planning, communication, and self-care, you can navigate social events successfully while managing your allergies.

Self-Care Practices For Managing Allergies

Self-care plays a crucial role in managing allergies and promoting overall well-being. Here are some self-care practices that can help you effectively cope with allergies:

Avoid Allergens: Identify and avoid your specific allergens as much as possible. This may involve staying indoors during high pollen or pollution days, keeping windows closed, using air purifiers, and taking precautions when in contact with known triggers.

Allergy-proof Your Home: Keep your living environment clean and free from allergens. Regularly dust and vacuum your home, use allergen-proof bedding covers, and consider using high-efficiency air filters to minimize indoor allergens.

Practice Good Hygiene: Practice good hygiene habits to reduce allergen exposure. Wash your hands frequently, especially after being outdoors, to remove allergens from your skin. Shower and change clothes after spending time outdoors to remove pollen or other allergens from your body and hair.

Maintain a Healthy Diet: Follow a balanced diet rich in nutrients to support your immune system and overall health. Incorporate foods that are known to have anti-inflammatory properties, such as fruits, vegetables, whole grains, and omega-3 fatty acids.

Stay Hydrated: Drink plenty of water to keep your body hydrated and support the natural functions of your respiratory system.

Manage Stress: Allergies can be exacerbated by stress, so it's important to manage stress levels. Engage in stress-reducing activities like exercise, meditation, deep breathing exercises, or hobbies that bring you joy and relaxation.

Get Regular Exercise: Regular physical activity can help boost your immune system and improve overall well-being. Choose activities that you enjoy and are suitable for your condition.

If exercising outdoors, be mindful of pollen counts and try to exercise when levels are lower.

Prioritize Sleep: Getting adequate sleep is essential for your overall health and immune system function. Create a sleep-friendly environment, establish a regular sleep schedule, and practice relaxation techniques before bed to promote restful sleep.

Use Saline Solutions: Rinsing your nasal passages with saline solutions can help alleviate nasal congestion and reduce allergy symptoms. Consider using a neti pot or nasal spray with a saline solution.

Seek Emotional Support: Allergies can have emotional impacts, so it's important to seek emotional support when needed. Reach out to loved ones, join support groups, or consider therapy or counseling to address any emotional challenges related to your allergies.

Remember, self-care practices may vary depending on your specific allergies and individual needs. It's important to work with your healthcare provider to develop a comprehensive self-care plan that suits your situation and supports your overall well-being.

Seeking Support And Building Resilience

Seeking support and building resilience are important aspects of managing allergies effectively. Here are some strategies to help you in this regard:

Seek Professional Support: Consult an allergist or immunologist who specializes in treating allergies. They can provide accurate diagnoses, offer personalized treatment plans, and guide you in managing your allergies effectively.

Join Allergy Support Groups: Connect with others who have similar allergies through support groups or online communities. Sharing experiences, tips, and advice can provide a sense of understanding and support.

Educate Yourself: Learn as much as you can about your allergies, triggers, and treatment options. Knowledge empowers you to make informed decisions and take control of your allergy management.

Communicate with Others: Inform your family, friends, colleagues, and others about your allergies. Let them know about your triggers and how they can help create an allergy-friendly environment when you are with them.

Practice Stress Management: Allergies can be stressful, so it's important to develop effective stress management techniques. Engage in activities that help you relax, such as deep breathing exercises, mindfulness meditation, yoga, or engaging in hobbies you enjoy.

Build Resilience: Develop resilience to cope with the challenges that allergies may bring. Focus on building a positive mindset, practicing gratitude, and finding meaning and purpose in your life. Surround yourself with a supportive network and seek help when needed.

Take Breaks When Needed: It's important to listen to your body and take breaks when necessary. If allergies are causing significant discomfort or fatigue, allow yourself time to rest and recharge.

Maintain a Balanced Lifestyle: Maintain a healthy and balanced lifestyle that includes proper nutrition, regular exercise, adequate sleep, and self-care practices. Taking care of your overall well-being can help strengthen your resilience and manage allergies more effectively.

Stay Positive and Flexible: Allergies can be unpredictable, so it's important to approach them with a positive and flexible mindset. Focus on what you can control and find alternative solutions or coping mechanisms when faced with challenges.

Celebrate Small Victories: Celebrate and acknowledge the progress you make in managing your allergies. Even small improvements or moments of relief should be recognized and celebrated as they contribute to your overall well-being.

Remember, seeking support and building resilience is an ongoing process. Be patient with yourself, and don't hesitate to reach out for help when needed. With the right support and resilience, you can effectively manage your allergies and lead a fulfilling life.

IX. Conclusion

Recap Of Allergy Relief Strategies

Here is a recap of the allergy relief strategies discussed:

Identify and avoid allergens: Determine your specific allergens and take steps to avoid them as much as possible.

Maintain a clean and allergy-friendly home environment: Regularly clean and dust your home, use allergen-proof bedding covers, and keep windows closed during peak allergy seasons.

Use over-the-counter medications: Antihistamines, decongestants, nasal sprays, and eye drops can provide temporary relief from allergy symptoms.

Consider natural remedies: Some people find relief with herbal remedies, such as butterbur, quercetin, or nettle leaf extract. Consult with a healthcare professional before using any natural remedies.

Try nasal rinses and saline sprays: These can help clear nasal passages and alleviate congestion.

Practice breathing exercises and relaxation techniques: Deep breathing exercises, meditation, and yoga can help reduce stress and manage allergy symptoms.

Explore essential oils: Certain essential oils, such as lavender, peppermint, and eucalyptus, may provide relief when used appropriately.

Seek prescription medications: If over-the-counter medications are not sufficient, your healthcare provider may prescribe stronger medications to manage your allergies.

Consider allergy shots (immunotherapy): Allergy shots can help desensitize your immune system to specific allergens and reduce your allergic response over time.

Take care of your overall health: Maintain a healthy lifestyle, including regular exercise, a balanced diet, adequate sleep, and proper hydration to support your immune system.

Create an allergy action plan: Work with your healthcare provider to develop an action plan that includes medication schedules, emergency contact information, and steps to take during an allergic reaction.

Seek support and resources: Join allergy support groups or seek information from reputable sources to learn from others' experiences and gain valuable tips.

Remember, it's important to consult with a healthcare professional for a proper diagnosis and personalized treatment plan. Allergy relief strategies may vary depending on individual circumstances, so it's essential to find what works best for you.

Encouragement For Readers On Their Allergy Journey

To all the readers on their allergy journey, I want to offer words of encouragement:

Living with allergies can be challenging, but you are not alone. Many people around the world face similar struggles, and there are resources and support available to help you navigate through it.

Remember that knowledge is power. Educate yourself about your specific allergies, triggers, and treatment options. Be proactive in seeking information and understanding your condition. This will empower you to make informed decisions and take necessary steps to manage your allergies effectively.

Stay resilient. Allergies can sometimes feel overwhelming, but you have the strength within you to overcome the challenges. Embrace a positive mindset, focus on what you can control, and celebrate even the small victories along the way.

Don't hesitate to seek support. Reach out to healthcare professionals, allergists, support groups, and online communities. Surround yourself with a network of people who understand and can provide guidance and encouragement. Share your experiences, ask questions, and learn from others who have walked a similar path.

Practice self-care. Taking care of yourself is crucial in managing allergies. Prioritize your well-being, both physically and emotionally. Engage in activities that bring you joy, reduce stress, and promote overall wellness. Remember to listen to your body and give it the rest, nourishment, and care it needs.

Lastly, be patient and compassionate with yourself. Managing allergies can be an ongoing process, and it may take time to find the right combination of strategies that work for you. Be kind to yourself during this journey, and remember that you are doing the best you can.

Keep exploring, learning, and adapting. With perseverance and determination, you can navigate your allergies and live a fulfilling life. Stay positive, stay informed, and know that you have the ability to overcome any challenges that come your way.

Wishing you strength, resilience, and improved well-being on your allergy journey.

Final Words Of Motivation And Empowerment

In closing, I want to leave you with these final words of motivation and empowerment:

You have the power to take control of your allergies and live a life that is not defined by them. You are stronger and more capable than you may realize. Embrace the challenges as opportunities for growth and resilience.

Remember that you are not defined by your allergies. They are just one aspect of your life. Focus on your strengths, passions, and the things that bring you joy. Let them be the driving force behind your journey.

Believe in yourself and your ability to overcome obstacles. Trust in your inner strength and the support systems you have in place. Surround yourself with positive influences, uplifting people, and resources that inspire and motivate you.

Keep learning and exploring. Stay curious about new treatments, strategies, and advancements in allergy management. Be open to trying different approaches and finding what works best for you.

Most importantly, be kind to yourself. Show yourself compassion, patience, and understanding as you navigate the ups and downs of managing allergies. Celebrate your progress, no matter how small, and give yourself permission to rest and recharge when needed.

You are not alone on this journey. There are countless others who have faced and overcome similar challenges. Seek out their stories, connect with them, and draw inspiration from their experiences.

Stay resilient, stay motivated, and stay empowered. Your journey is unique, and you have the strength to navigate it with grace and determination. Trust in yourself, believe in your abilities, and embrace the possibilities that lie ahead.

May you find comfort, relief, and empowerment on your allergy journey. Keep moving forward, and remember that you are capable of creating a life filled with health, happiness, and fulfillment.

Additional Resources And References For Further Exploration

Here are some additional resources and references that you can explore for further information on allergies:

American Academy of Allergy, Asthma & Immunology (AAAAI): Provides comprehensive information on allergies, asthma, and immunology. Website: https://www.aaaai.org/

Allergy and Asthma Foundation of America (AAFA): Offers resources, education, and support for individuals with allergies and asthma. Website: https://www.aafa.org/

Mayo Clinic: Provides reliable and up-to-date information on various health topics, including allergies. Website: https://www.mayoclinic.org/

National Institute of Allergy and Infectious Diseases (NIAID): Conducts research and provides resources on allergies, immunology, and related topics. Website: https://www.niaid.nih.gov/

Asthma and Allergy Foundation of America (AAFA): Offers educational resources, support, and advocacy for individuals with allergies and asthma. Website: https://www.aafa.org/

Allergy UK: Provides information and support for people with allergies, including resources on allergy management and living with allergies. Website: https://www.allergyuk.org/

Food Allergy Research & Education (FARE): Focuses on food allergies and provides resources, support, and advocacy for individuals and families affected by food allergies. Website: https://www.foodallergy.org/

Allergic Living: A magazine and online resource providing information, articles, and tips on living with allergies and related conditions. Website: https://www.allergicliving.com/

These resources offer a wealth of information, support, and guidance for individuals dealing with allergies. They cover various aspects of allergies, including management, prevention, treatment options, and lifestyle considerations. Additionally, consulting with healthcare professionals, such as allergists and immunologists, can provide personalized advice and guidance tailored to your specific needs.

Remember to always consult with a healthcare professional for accurate diagnosis, treatment options, and personalized advice regarding your specific allergy condition.

Wishing you all the best in your journey towards allergy management and well-being!